Student's Manual
MBBS FOUNDATION COURSE

Student's Manual
MBBS FOUNDATION COURSE

Competency-based Medical Curriculum

Manisha Jindal MBBS MD DFM
Professor Physiology
Dean
School of Medical Sciences and Research
Sharda University
Greater Noida, Uttar Pradesh, India

JAYPEE
JAYPEE BROTHERS MEDICAL PUBLISHERS
The Health Sciences Publisher
New Delhi | London

Jaypee Brothers Medical Publishers (P) Ltd

Headquarters
EMCA House, 23/23-B
Ansari Road, Daryaganj
New Delhi 110 002, India
Landline: +91-11-23272143, +91-11-23272703
+91-11-23282021, +91-11-23245672
e-mail: jaypee@jaypeebrothers.com

Corporate Office
4838/24, Ansari Road, Daryaganj
New Delhi 110 002, India
Phone: +91-11-43574357
Fax: +91-11-43574314
e-mail: jaypee@jaypeebrothers.com

Overseas Office
JP Medical Ltd.
83, Victoria Street, London
SW1H 0HW (UK)
Phone: +44-20 3170 8910
e-mail: info@jpmedpub.com

EU GPSR Authorised Representative
Logos Europe, 9 rue Nicolas Poussin
17000, La Rochelle, France
Phone: +33 (0) 6 67 93 73 78
e-mail: contact@logoseurope.eu

Website: www.jaypeebrothers.com
Website: www.jaypeedigital.com

Inquiries for bulk sales may be solicited at: jaypee@jaypeebrothers.com

Student's Manual MBBS Foundation Course

First Edition: **2022**

Reprint: **2025**

ISBN: 978-93-5465-185-4

Printed in India at Purewall Ventures Pvt Ltd

Preface

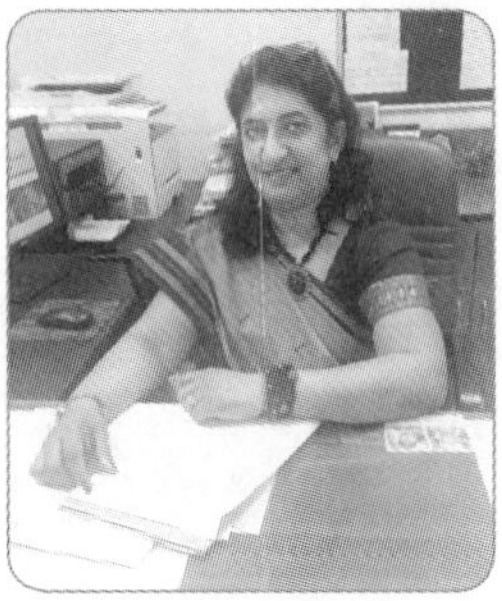

The new competency-based medical education (CBME) curriculum advised by the Board of Governors in supersession of MCI has been a novel step in ensuring standardized and good medical education to our budding doctors.

The concept of foundation course is an innovative plan for ensuring that all students entering the medical undergraduate program come at par with each other and have the prerequisite awareness and knowledge about the basics of the curriculum in addition to providing valuable guidance regarding participation in sports and other extracurricular activities.

Each of the domains in the foundation course will be adding value to the learning of the medical undergraduate and sensitizing him/her in respect of orientation to the medical school and program, basic essential skills and their development, community and field visits, professionalism and ethics, sports and extracurricular activities as well as computer skills. Many of these were earlier a part of the hidden curricula, which was never emphasized and, hence, never optimally understood leading to several lacunae.

This logbook enables the learner to maintain a record of the daily activities and also provides the faculty member adequate feedback of how successful the teaching learning during foundation course has been. It ensures proper concept building in the mind of the student. Each module has the objectives prescribed by the governing council and is divided into subsections followed by an assessment in the form of short answer questions in addition to providing the guidelines for conduction of that module as prescribed by the Board of Governors in supersession of MCI.

I hope that both the students and the faculty members will find this logbook useful in the initial formative one month of the MBBS program.

Manisha Jindal

Contents

Introduction

OBJECTIVE OF THE COURSE

The objective of this one-month duration **Foundation Course** at the beginning of the MBBS course is to sensitize the fresh medical student with the required knowledge and skills that will assist him/her in acclimatizing to the new professional environment which would be his/her milieu for a life-long career in the medical profession. The Foundation Course will also provide a sound foundation for learning in the MBBS course and later in their professional career.

Glossary of Terms Used in the Document

Orientation: Refers to the awareness created in new students with respect to place (learning environment and facility), time, teaching schedules and time-tables, processes (rules, regulations, policies and procedures), personnel (faculty, staff, and mentors), patients and their relatives.

Skills Module: Refers to basic skills that are considered important for all healthcare personnel who deal with patients and requires students to be trained in prior to entering patientcare areas.

Enhancement skills: Refers to those skills which are needed to enable students from diverse backgrounds (including different boards, language of instruction, culture and varied degrees of technological exposure) to appreciate and accommodate the similarities and differences in medical practice and to feel at par with each other.

Sports and extracurricular activities: Refers to sports and extracurricular activities permitted within the time schedule.

Professionalism and ethics: Professionalism defines a set of values and behavior that build the trust that a patient has on his/her doctor. Ethics are principles that govern the behavior of doctors. Professional competence, effective communication and ethics are the three founding principles of Professionalism.

Introduction

Medical education in India requires training in a wide spectrum of domains that involves exposure to human interactions and interpersonal relationships in various settings including hospital, community, clinics, etc. The training is intense and demands great commitment, resilience and lifelong learning. Students enter in a new environment in medical college at around 17 years of age directly from school which can be challenging. Therefore, it is desirable to create a period of acclimatization and familiarization to the new environment. This would include an introduction to the course structure, learning methods, technology usage, and peer interactions which would facilitate their smooth transition from high school to medical college.

This is proposed to be achieved through a dedicated one month exclusive "Foundation Course", at the beginning of the MBBS course, to orient and sensitize the student to the various identified areas. Many of these identified areas will need to be followed up by more focused outcome-based sessions at various stages in the MBBS course. This will be achieved through activities/small courses integrated throughout the course which will be like the thread running through a garland. At appropriate stages throughout the course, emphasis will be laid on the various essential roles of the "Indian Medical Graduate".

Purpose

The purpose of the Foundation Course include:
- Orienting the students to all aspects of the medical college environment.
- Equipping them with certain basic, but important, skills required for patient care and enhancing their communication, language, computer and learning skills.
- Providing opportunity for peer and faculty interactions and an overall sensitization to the various learning methodologies.

Context from proposed GMER Graduate Medical Education Regulations) 2019

Foundation Course

Goal: The goal of the Foundation Course is to prepare a learner to study Medicine effectively. It will be of one-month duration after admission.
- **Objectives:** The objectives are to:
  - **Orient the learner to:**
    - The medical profession and the physician's role in society
    - The MBBS program
    - Alternate health systems in the country and history of medicine
    - Medical ethics, attitudes and professionalism
    - Healthcare system and its delivery
    - National health priorities and policies

    - Universal precautions and vaccinations
    - Patient safety and biohazard safety
    - Principles of primary care (general and community-based care)
    - The academic ambience
  - **Enable the learner to acquire enhanced skills in:**
    - Language
    - Interpersonal relationships
    - Communication
    - Learning including self-directed learning
    - Time management
    - Stress management
    - Use of information technology
  - **Train the learner to provide:**
    - First-aid
    - Basic life support
- In addition to the above, learners may be enrolled in one of the following programs which will be run concurrently:
  - Local language program
  - English language program
  - Computer skills
- These sessions will be as interactive as possible.

STRUCTURE OF THE PROGRAM FOR STUDENTS	
Subjects/Contents	*Total Teaching hours*
1. Orientation	30
2. Skills Module	35
3. Field visit to community health center	8
4. Professional development including ethics	40
5. Enhancement of language/computer skills	40
6. Sports and extracurricular activities	22
Total teaching hours	**175**

Sports will be for a mandatory 4 hours per week and extracurricular activities 2 hours per week, subject to a total of 22 hours.

LEARNING OUTCOMES

Code	*COMPETENCY* *The student should be able to:*	Domain	K/KH/SH/P
1	***Orientation***		
FC 1.1	Demonstrate understanding of the role of doctors in the society and their impact	A	KH
FC 1.2	Demonstrate understanding of the roles of an Indian Medical Graduate and relate it to the societal impact	A	KH
FC 1.3	Discuss and appreciate the expectations of the students from the nation, society, institution, peers, colleagues and patients and vice versa	A	KH
FC 1.4	Demonstrate understanding of the rules and regulations of the institution	A	SH
FC 1.5	Orient themselves to the college campus, facilities, faculty, administrative structure, support systems and processes of the institution	A	KH
FC 1.6	Discuss the various career pathways and opportunities for personal growth	A	KH
FC 1.7	Demonstrate understanding of the overview of MBBS curriculum, its structure and outcomes and its relation to the career pathways	K	KH
FC 1.8	Demonstrate understanding the role of physician at various levels of healthcare delivery	K	KH
FC 1.9	Discuss the principles of family practice	K	KH
FC 1.10	Demonstrate awareness of the History of Medicine and alternate systems of Medicine	K	K
2	***Skills***		
FC 2.1	Perform basic life support in skills lab	S	SH
FC 2.2	Perform first aid in a simulated environment	S	SH
FC 2.3	Follow biosafety and universal precautions	S	SH
FC 2.4	Demonstrate handling and safe disposal of biohazardous materials in a simulated environment	S	SH
FC 2.5	Demonstrate proper hand washing and use of personal protective equipment	S	SH

FC 2.6	Demonstrate appropriate response to needle stick injuries	S	SH
FC 2.7	Demonstrate Biomedical Waste (BMW) segregation, observe and explain the process of management of BMW in accordance with National Regulations	S	SH
FC 2.8	Discuss the immunization requirements of health care professionals	K	KH
FC 2.9	Demonstrate awareness of significance of documentation in patient care and the proper method of documentation	S	SH
3	***Community orientation and field visits***		
FC 3.1	Demonstrate understanding of the National Health Goals and Policies	K	KH
FC 3.2	Discuss the national health scenario, demographic, socio-cultural and epidemiological issues	K	KH
FC 3.3	Demonstrate understanding of the health care systems in India with reference to primary, secondary and tertiary level care	K	KH
FC 3.4	Discuss the basic principles of community health and its impact on health and disease	S	SH
FC 3.5	Demonstrate understanding of the structure and functioning of the community health center	K	KH
FC 3.6	Demonstrate ability to obtain patient experiences through patient and family interactions and relate these experiences to impact of environment and diseases	S	SH
4	***Professional development including ethics***		
FC 4.1	Demonstrate understanding of the concept of professionalism and ethics among health care professionals and discuss the consequences of unprofessional and unethical behavior	S	KH
FC 4.2	Demonstrate understanding that compassion, altruism, integrity, duty, responsibility and trust are the core values that defines the nature of the physician's work	K	KH
FC 4.3	Discuss the value, honesty and respect during interaction with peers, seniors, faculty, other health care workers and patients	S	KH
FC 4.4	Discuss the significance of working in a health care team	S	KH
FC 4.5	Discuss disability competencies	K	KH

FC 4.6	Demonstrate understanding and respect of cultural diversities and interact with those with different cultural values	K/A	KH
FC 4.7	Discuss the significance and methods of stress management and risk taking behavior	K	KH
FC 4.8	Understand the role of yoga and meditation in personal health	S	S
FC 4.9	Discuss the significance and appropriate ways of time management	K	KH
FC 4.10	Demonstrate understanding of importance of interpersonal relationship while working in a health care team	S	KH
FC 4.11	Understand the role of mentoring	S	KH
FC 4.12	Demonstrates understanding of the process of group learning and group dynamics	S	KH
FC 4.13	Comprehend the learning pedagogy and its role in learning skills	S	KH
FC 4.14	Demonstrates understanding of different methods of self-directed learning	S	KH
FC 4.15	Understand collaborative learning	S	KH
5	***Enhancement skills—communication and language skills***		
FC 5.1	Demonstrate ability to communicate with patient and families, be aware of barriers to communication and appropriate ways to respond	C	SH
FC 5.2	Demonstrate use of local language in patient and peer interactions	C	SH
FC 5.3	Demonstrate ability to communicate and learn in English	C	SH
FC 5.4	Demonstrate basic computer skills	S	SH
FC 5.5	Demonstrate ability for accessing online resources	S	SH

1

Orientation

Duration: 30 hours

LEARNING OUTCOMES: ORIENTATION

Code	*COMPETENCY* *The student should be able to:*	Domain	K/KH/SH/P
FC 1.1	Demonstrate understanding of the role of doctors in the society and their impact	A	KH
FC 1.2	Demonstrate understanding of the roles of an Indian Medical Graduate and relate it to the societal impact	A	KH
FC 1.3	Discuss and appreciate the expectations of the students from the nation, society, institution, peers, colleagues and patients and vice versa	A	KH
FC 1.4	Demonstrate understanding of the rules and regulations of the institution	A	SH
FC 1.5	Orient themselves to the college campus, facilities, faculty, administrative structure, support systems and processes of the institution	A	KH
FC 1.6	Discuss the various career pathways and opportunities for personal growth	A	KH
FC 1.7	Demonstrate understanding of the overview of MBBS curriculum, its structure and outcomes and its relation to the career pathways	K	KH
FC 1.8	Demonstrate understanding the role of physician at various levels of health care delivery	K	KH
FC 1.9	Discuss the principles of family practice	K	KH
FC 1.10	Demonstrate awareness of the history of medicine and alternate systems of medicine	K	K

1.1 ORIENTATION: INTRODUCTION TO INSTITUTION/CAMPUS FACILITIES

Date:.................... **Time:............** **Duration:.........................**

Learning objectives of the module:

TEACHING LEARNING METHODOLOGY

No.	*Content area*	*Methodology*	*Time*	*Remarks of student*
1.	Welcome and Introduction by Institutional heads	Inspiring talk… to the new MBBS graduates and their parents	2 hours	
2.	Understanding Vision/Mission of the institution			
3.	Understanding Roles of an Indian Medical Graduate			
4.	Expectation of the students from Nation, Society, Institutions, colleagues and peers	Overview lecture/interactive discussion	1 hour	
5.	Rules and Regulations of the institution	Overview lecture/interactive discussion	1 hour	
6.	Orientation to the college/campus/ facilities	Walk through the college including lecture halls, common rooms, preclinical departments, office of the Dean and administration, library, food facilities, security facilities, auditorium—mini talks at important facilities regarding Rules and Regulations	4 hours	
7.	Introduction to faculty/mentors	Interactive session with faculty mentors and peers	2 hours	

1.1 ASSESSMENT: INTRODUCTION TO INSTITUTION/CAMPUS FACILITIES

1. State 5 important rules and regulations of your institute.

2. What is the vision of your institute?

3. What do you like about your institution at a glance?

4. What are the chief take home points in the talks given to you today?

1.2 ORIENTATION: ROLE OF DOCTORS IN SOCIETY

Date:.................... **Time:............** **Duration:........................**

Learning objectives of the module:

Teaching learning methodology:

1.2 ASSESSMENT: ROLE OF DOCTORS IN SOCIETY

1. What is your perception of roles of doctors at various levels of health care delivery?

2. What was your main motivation to join the medical profession?

3. Do doctors have privileged roles in society that they can exploit for greater common good?

4. What according to you are the major limitations for optimal performance of doctors?

1.3 ORIENTATION: HISTORY OF MEDICINE AND ALTERNATE SYSTEMS

Date:.................... **Time:............** **Duration:........................**

Learning objectives of the module:

Teaching learning methodology:

1.3 ASSESSMENT: HISTORY OF MEDICINE AND ALTERNATE SYSTEMS

1. What is alternative medicine?

2. What is complementary medicine?

3. What is evidence-based medicine?

4. What is the difference between modern medicine and complementary and alternative medicine (CAM)?

5. What according to you is practice impact?

1.4 ORIENTATION: ROLES OF IMG, OVERVIEW OF MEDICAL CURRICULUM AND CAREER PATHWAYS

Date:.................... **Time:............** **Duration:........................**

Learning objectives of the module:

Teaching learning methodology:

1.4 ASSESSMENT: ROLES OF IMG, OVERVIEW OF MEDICAL CURRICULUM AND CAREER PATHWAYS

1. Reflect on the roles of Indian medical graduate and relate it to societal impact.

2. Discuss the significance of 'competency based medical curriculum'.

3. What are the various career pathways available for your personal growth?

4. Discuss the structure of the MBBS Program?

1.5 ORIENTATION: PRINCIPLES OF FAMILY PRACTICE

Date:.................... **Time:............** **Duration:........................**

Learning objectives of the module:

Teaching learning methodology:

1.5 ASSESSMENT: PRINCIPLES OF FAMILY PRACTICE

1. What is your perception of roles of physician at various levels of health care delivery?

2. State in your words the principles of family practice.

2

Skills Module

Duration: 35 hours

LEARNING OUTCOMES: SKILLS MODULE

Code	*COMPETENCY* *The student should be able to:*	*Domain*	*K/KH/SH/P*
FC 2.1	Perform Basic Life support in Skills lab	S	SH
FC 2.2	Perform First Aid in a simulated environment	S	SH
FC 2.3	Follow bio-safety and universal precautions	S	SH
FC 2.4	Demonstrate handling and safe disposal of biohazardous materials in a simulated environment	S	SH
FC 2.5	Demonstrate proper hand washing and use of personal protective equipment	S	SH
FC 2.6	Demonstrate appropriate response to needle stick injuries	S	SH
FC 2.7	Demonstrate Biomedical Waste (BMW) segregation, observe and explain the process of management of BMW in accordance with National Regulations	S	SH
FC 2.8	Discuss the immunization requirements of health care professionals	K	KH
FC 2.9	Demonstrate awareness of significance of documentation in patient care and the proper method of documentation	S	SH

2.1 SKILLS: BASIC LIFE SUPPORT

Date:.................... **Time:............** **Duration:.........................**

Learning objectives of the module:

Teaching learning methodology:

2.1 ASSESSMENT: BASIC LIFE SUPPORT

Perform 'Basic Life support' in Skills lab

The student can perform 'Basic Life support'.

Certified by ....

Signature and Date.....................................

1. What are the different components of Basic Life Support?

2. In which conditions would you require your skills for Basic Life support?

Learning objectives of the module:

3. How would acquisition of this skill aid you in becoming a better doctor?

2.2 SKILLS: FIRST AID

Date:.................... **Time:............** **Duration:.........................**

Learning objectives of the module:

Teaching learning methodology:

2.2 ASSESSMENT: FIRST AID

Perform 'First Aid' in a simulated environment.

The student can perform 'First Aid' in a simulated environment.

Certified by ....

Signature and Date.....................................

1. Tabulate the appropriate first aid methods that would be needed in 5 different life-threatening emergency situations

No.	*Life-threatening situations*	*Appropriate first aid method*
1.		
2.		
3.		
4.		
5.		

2.3 SKILLS: UNIVERSAL PRECAUTIONS

Date:.................... **Time:............** **Duration:........................**

Learning objectives of the module:

Teaching learning methodology:

2.3 ASSESSMENT: UNIVERSAL PRECAUTIONS

Demonstrate proper hand washing and use of personal protective equipment (PPE)

The student can demonstrate proper hand washing and use of PPE.

Certified by ....

Signature and Date....................................

1. Define universal precautions.

2. List essential components of universal precautions.

3. List infective and non-infective body fluids.

4. Discuss appropriate response to needle stick injuries.

2.4 SKILLS: WASTE MANAGEMENT

Date:.................. **Time:...........** **Duration:......................**

Learning objectives of the module:

Teaching learning methodology:

2.4 ASSESSMENT: WASTE MANAGEMENT

Demonstrate proper segregation of biomedical waste.

The student can demonstrate proper segregation of biomedical waste.

Certified by ....

Signature and Date....................................

1. Define biomedical waste.

2. List different types of waste generated in a health care facility.

3. Explain the hazards of improper disposal of biomedical waste.

4. How can waste be segregated?

5. How can biomedical waste be disposed?

2.5 SKILLS: IMMUNIZATION

Date:.................. **Time:...........** **Duration:.......................**

Learning objectives of the module:

Teaching learning methodology:

2.5 ASSESSMENT: IMMUNIZATION

1. What do you understand by the term 'immunization'?

2. List the vaccine preventable diseases.

3. Why is vaccination important for staff and students?

4. Discuss the vaccination recommendation for health care personnel.

2.6 SKILLS : DOCUMENTATION

Date:.................. **Time:...........** **Duration:.......................**

Learning objectives of the module:

Teaching learning methodology:

2.6 ASSESSMENT: DOCUMENTATION

1. Explain the importance of documentation as a doctor.

2. Discuss the consequences of appropriate and inappropriate documentation on the safety of patient.

3

Community Health and Field Visits

Duration: 8 hours

LEARNING OUTCOMES: COMMUNITY ORIENTATION AND FIELD VISITS

Code	*COMPETENCY* *The student should be able to:*	*Domain*	*K/KH/SH/P*
FC 3.1	Demonstrate understanding of the national health goals and policies	K	KH
FC 3.2	Discuss the national health scenario, demographic, socio-cultural and epidemiological issues	K	KH
FC 3.3	Demonstrate understanding of the health care systems in India with reference to primary, secondary and tertiary level care	K	KH
FC 3.4	Discuss the basic principles of community health and its impact on health and disease	S	SH
FC 3.5	Demonstrate understanding of the structure and functioning of the community health center	K	KH
FC 3.6	Demonstrate ability to obtain patient experiences through patient and family interactions and relate these experiences to impact of environment and diseases	S	SH

3.1 COMMUNITY ORIENTATION: NATIONAL HEALTH GOALS AND POLICIES

Date:.................... **Time:............** **Duration:........................**

Learning objectives of the module:

Teaching learning methodology:

3.1 ASSESSMENT: NATIONAL HEALTH GOALS AND POLICIES

1. Give your reflection on the national health scenario in context of socio-cultural, demographic and ethical issues.

2. Discuss the health care system in India at primary, secondary and tertiary care level.

3. Discuss the basic principles of community health and its impact on health and disease.

3.2 COMMUNITY ORIENTATION: INTERACTIONS WITH PATIENTS AND FAMILIES IN COMMUNITY

Date:.................... **Time:............** **Duration:........................**

Learning objectives of the module:

Teaching learning methodology:

Community site visited and its location:

3.2 ASSESSMENT: INTERACTIONS WITH PATIENTS AND FAMILIES IN COMMUNITY

1. Give your reflection on the effect of family and social environment in the etiology of diseases.

2. Comment on the environmental health problems in the community.

3. List some common community beliefs and practices related to health and diseases.

4

Professional Development and Ethics

Duration: 40 hours

LEARNING OUTCOMES: PROFESSIONAL DEVELOPMENT INCLUDING ETHICS

Code	*COMPETENCY* *The student should be able to:*	*Domain*	*K/KH/SH/P*
FC 4.1	Demonstrate understanding of the concept of Professionalism and ethics among health care professionals and discuss the consequences of unprofessional and unethical behavior	S	KH
FC 4.2	Demonstrate understanding that compassion, altruism, integrity, duty, responsibility and trust are the core values that defines the nature of the physician's work	K	KH
FC 4.3	Discuss the value, honesty and respect during interaction with peers, seniors, faculty, other health care workers and patients	S	KH
FC 4.4	Discuss the significance of working in a health care team	S	KH
FC 4.5	Discuss disability competencies	K	KH
FC 4.6	Demonstrate understanding and respect of cultural diversities and interact with those with different cultural values	K/A	KH
FC 4.7	Discuss the significance and methods of stress management and risk taking behavior	K	KH
FC 4.8	Understand the role of yoga and meditation in personal health	S	S
FC 4.9	Discuss the significance and appropriate ways of time management	K	KH
FC 4.10	Demonstrate understanding of importance of interpersonal relationship while working in a health care team	S	KH
FC 4.11	Understand the role of mentoring	S	KH
FC 4.12	Demonstrates understanding of the process of group learning and group dynamics	S	KH
FC 4.13	Comprehend the learning pedagogy and its role in learning skills	S	KH
FC 4.14	Demonstrates understanding of different methods of self-directed learning	S	KH
FC 4.15	Understand collaborative learning	S	KH

4.1 PROFESSIONAL DEVELOPMENT: CONCEPT OF PROFESSIONALISM AND ETHICS

Date:.................... **Time:............** **Duration:........................**

Learning objectives of the module:

Teaching learning methodology:

4.1 ASSESSMENT: CONCEPT OF PROFESSIONALISM AND ETHICS

1. Why is professionalism important in health care professionals?

2. List some unprofessional/unethical practices that some medical professionals follow.

3. Reflect on the consequences of unethical behavior by a doctor.

4.2 PROFESSIONAL DEVELOPMENT: WHITE COAT CEREMONY

Date:.................... **Time:............** **Duration:........................**

Learning objectives of the module:

Teaching learning methodology:

4.2 ASSESSMENT: WHITE COAT CEREMONY

1. Give your reflections on the significance of white coat ceremony.

4.3 PROFESSIONAL DEVELOPMENT: PROFESSIONAL AND ALTRUISTIC BEHAVIOR

Date:................... **Time:...........** **Duration:.......................**

Learning objectives of the module:

Teaching learning methodology:

4.3 ASSESSMENT: PROFESSIONAL AND ALTRUISTIC BEHAVIOR

1. Define altruism.

2. Give your reflections on why altruism is a core virtue of a physician.

4.4 PROFESSIONAL DEVELOPMENT: WORKING IN A HEALTH CARE TEAM

Date:.................... **Time:............** **Duration:.........................**

Learning objectives of the module:

Teaching learning methodology:

4.4 ASSESSMENT: WORKING IN A HEALTH CARE TEAM

1. What is the difference between a 'team' and a 'group'?

2. What are the important aspects required to build a good team?

3. Discuss the role of honesty, respect and trust in a 'team'.

4.5 PROFESSIONAL DEVELOPMENT: DISABILITY COMPETENCIES

Date:.................. **Time:...........** **Duration:.......................**

Learning objectives of the module:

Teaching learning methodology:

4.5 ASSESSMENT: DISABILITY COMPETENCIES

1. Describe 'disability' as per UN convention on the rights of persons with disabilities'.

2. Compare and contrast the medical and social model of disability.

3. List some 'disability friendly' modifications that are available in your institute.

4.6 PROFESSIONAL DEVELOPMENT: CULTURAL COMPETENCE

Date:.................... **Time:............** **Duration:.........................**

Learning objectives of the module:

Teaching learning methodology:

4.6 ASSESSMENT: CULTURAL COMPETENCE

1. What do you understand by the term 'cultural competence'?

2. Describe the components of cultural competence.

3. How would cultural competency help you in becoming a better medical professional?

4.7 PROFESSIONAL DEVELOPMENT: STRESS MANAGEMENT

Date:.................... **Time:............** **Duration:.........................**

Learning objectives of the module:

Teaching learning methodology:

4.7 ASSESSMENT: STRESS MANAGEMENT

1. How do you define stress?

2. What according to you are the major stressors in learning period of a budding doctor?

3. Discuss the health impact of stress.

4. Give your views on the various stress management techniques.

4.8 PROFESSIONAL DEVELOPMENT: TIME MANAGEMENT

Date:................... **Time:...........** **Duration:.......................**

Learning objectives of the module:

Teaching learning methodology:

4.8 ASSESSMENT: TIME MANAGEMENT

1. Describe the importance of time management.

2. List some of the common distractions that would deter you from effective time management.

3. Make a schedule of your typical weekday as a learner to manage time effectively.

No.	*Time/ Duration*	*Activity*	*Remarks*

4.9 PROFESSIONAL DEVELOPMENT: INTERPERSONAL RELATIONSHIP

Date:.................... **Time:............** **Duration:........................**

Learning objectives of the module:

Teaching learning methodology:

4.9 ASSESSMENT: INTERPERSONAL RELATIONSHIP

1. Give your reflection on the importance of good interpersonal relationship for a medical professional.

2. What are the roles and responsibilities of the mentee.

3. List some barriers in formation of good interpersonal relationships.

4.10 PROFESSIONAL DEVELOPMENT: LEARNING

Date:.................... **Time:............** **Duration:........................**

Learning objectives of the module:

Teaching learning methodology:

4.10 ASSESSMENT: LEARNING

1. What are the advantages of didactic method of teaching learning?

2. List some advantages of small group teaching learning.

3. List some methods of self-directed learning and their advantages.

4. What is collaborative learning? Give its importance.

5

Enhancement of Language and Computer Skills

Duration: 40 hours

LEARNING OUTCOMES: ENHANCEMENT OF LANGUAGE AND COMPUTER SKILLS

Code	*COMPETENCY* *The student should be able to:*	*Domain*	*K/KH/SH/P*
FC 5.1	Demonstrate ability to communicate with patient and families, be aware of barriers to communication and appropriate ways to respond	C	SH
FC 5.2	Demonstrate use of local language in patient and peer interactions	C	SH
FC 5.3	Demonstrate ability to communicate and learn in English	C	SH
FC 5.4	Demonstrate basic computer skills	S	SH
FC 5.5	Demonstrate ability for accessing online resources	S	SH

5.1 ENHANCEMENT OF LANGUAGE AND COMPUTER SKILLS: COMMUNICATION PROFESSIONAL AND ALTRUISTIC BEHAVIOR

Date:.................... **Time:............** **Duration:........................**

Learning objectives of the module:

Teaching learning methodology:

5.1 ASSESSMENT: COMMUNICATION

1. Give your reflection on the importance of good communication skills for a health care professional.

2. List the barriers for good communication.

3. What is the difference between:

i. Hearing and listening

ii. Empathy and sympathy

5.2 AND 5.3 ENHANCEMENT SKILLS MODULE: LOCAL LANGUAGE AND ENGLISH LANGUAGE SKILLS

Date:.................... **Time:............** **Duration:........................**

Learning objectives of the module:

Teaching learning methodology:

5.2 AND 5.3 ASSESSMENT: LOCAL LANGUAGE AND ENGLISH LANGUAGE SKILLS

1. How would knowledge of local language be helpful in becoming a better clinician?

2. Give your reflections on 'Why having knowledge of English language' may help you in becoming a better doctor.

5.4 ENHANCEMENT SKILLS MODULE: BASIC COMPUTER SKILLS

Date:.................... **Time:............** **Duration:........................**

Learning objectives of the module:

Teaching learning methodology:

5.4 ASSESSMENT: BASIC COMPUTER SKILLS

1. Why do you think basic knowledge of computers will assist you in becoming a better clinician?

2. List your strengths and weaknesses in using computer knowledge for advanced teaching learning.

3. List some online learning apps/platforms that you can use for facilitating teaching learning via mobiles or computers.

4. What is e-learning?

6

Sports and Extracurricular Activities

Duration: 22 hours

Learning objectives of the module:

Tabulate your involvement in the various sports and extracurricular activities that you participated during Foundation course

S. No.	*Activity*	*Duration*

DISCUSSION: SPORTS AND EXTRACURRICULAR ACTIVITIES

1. Which sports activities are you good at?

2. List the different extracurricular activities that you have participated in till your class 12th.

3. Why are sports and extracurricular activities in your life as a learner?

7

History of Outbreaks, Epidemics and Pandemics

Duration: 2 hours

Date:..................... **Time:............** **Duration:.........................**

Learning objectives of the module:

Tabulate five major pandemics that have caused a major health hazard in the history.

S. No.	*Pandemic*	*Timeline and Duration*

DISCUSSION: COVID-19

1. What is the full form of COVID-19?

2. What was the causative organism?

3. What was the mode of transmission?

4. List the main clinical presentation of COVID-19 and the major cause of death.

5. What preventive measures were advised to contain the spread of virus?

Final Summary of Foundation Course

S. No.	*Module*	*Date*		*Attendance*	*Status Complete / incomplete*	*Sign of teacher*
		To	*From*			
1.						
2.						
3.						
4.						
5.						
6.						
7.						

References

1. Module 1- Foundation Course for the Undergraduate Medical Education Program, 2019, Board of Governors in supersession of MCI.
2. Module 7- Module on Pandemic Management, August 2020, Board of Governors in supersession of MCI.

Student's Name: ....

Roll No. ....

Year of Admission: ....

Name of Institution: ....

University to which Institute Affiliated: ....

....

....

....

....

It is hereby certified that this logbook has been completed by the student .... in the month of .... Year ....The skills have been verified by faculty in-charge.

Signature of Co-ordinator

Signature of Dean

Student name: ....

....

Internal Institution ....

It is hereby certified that all the practicals were completed by the student

.... in the month of ....

Year .... The files have been certified by the faculty ....

Signature of Dean